Cambridge Elements ≡

Elements in Emergency Neurosurgery
edited by
Nihal Gurusinghe
Lancashire Teaching Hospital NHS Trust
Peter Hutchinson
University of Cambridge, Society of British Neurological Surgeons and Royal College of Surgeons of England
Ioannis Fouyas
Royal College of Surgeons of Edinburgh
Naomi Slator
North Bristol NHS Trust
Ian Kamaly-Asl
Royal Manchester Children's Hospital
Peter Whitfield
University Hospitals Plymouth NHS Trust

MODELS FOR DELIVERING HIGH QUALITY EMERGENCY NEUROSURGERY IN HIGH INCOME COUNTRIES

Matthew A. Boissaud-Cooke
University Hospitals Plymouth NHS Trust
Marike Broekman
Leiden University Medical Centre
Jeroen van Dijck
Leiden University Medical Centre
Marco Lee
Stanford Department of Neurosurgery
Paul Grundy
University Hospital Southampton

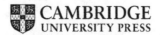

CAMBRIDGE
UNIVERSITY PRESS

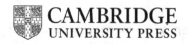

CAMBRIDGE
UNIVERSITY PRESS

Shaftesbury Road, Cambridge CB2 8EA, United Kingdom

One Liberty Plaza, 20th Floor, New York, NY 10006, USA

477 Williamstown Road, Port Melbourne, VIC 3207, Australia

314–321, 3rd Floor, Plot 3, Splendor Forum, Jasola District Centre, New Delhi – 110025, India

103 Penang Road, #05–06/07, Visioncrest Commercial, Singapore 238467

Cambridge University Press is part of Cambridge University Press & Assessment, a department of the University of Cambridge.

We share the University's mission to contribute to society through the pursuit of education, learning and research at the highest international levels of excellence.

www.cambridge.org
Information on this title: www.cambridge.org/9781009478830

DOI: 10.1017/9781009366113

First published 2024

A catalogue record for this publication is available from the British Library

ISBN 978-1-009-47883-0 Hardback
ISBN 978-1-009-36610-6 Paperback
ISSN 2755-0656 (online)
ISSN 2755-0648 (print)

Models for Delivering High Quality Emergency Neurosurgery in High Income Countries

Elements in Emergency Neurosurgery

DOI: 10.1017/9781009366113
First published online: January 2024

Matthew A. Boissaud-Cooke
University Hospitals Plymouth NHS Trust

Marike Broekman
Leiden University Medical Centre

Jeroen van Dijck
Leiden University Medical Centre

Marco Lee
Stanford Department of Neurosurgery

Paul Grundy
University Hospital Southampton

Author for correspondence: Matthew A. Boissaud-Cooke,
Matthew.boissaud-cooke@nhs.net

Abstract: Emergency neurosurgery encompasses serious and high-risk cranial and spinal conditions across all ages. The authors provide an overview of the changes occurring within emergency surgery to meet the challenges provided from unscheduled care. Considering the wider landscape of emergency surgery provides a context for the changes occurring within emergency neurosurgery. The delivery of emergency neurosurgery within the UK, the Republic of Ireland, the Netherlands and the United States of America is then described to provide an overview of different models of care.

Keywords: unscheduled care, emergency surgery, emergency neurosurgery, high quality, emergency

ISBNs: 9781009478830 (HB), 9781009366106 (PB), 9781009366113 (OC)
ISSNs: 2755-0656 (online), 2755-0648 (print)

Contents

Introduction

The World Health Organisation considers the quality of care as 'the degree to which health services for individuals and people increase the likelihood of desired health outcomes and are consistent with evidence-based professional knowledge'. Health services strive to deliver the highest quality of healthcare determined by the resources available to them. The delivery of high-quality emergency (neuro)surgery is fraught with difficulty requiring the optimising of services that must respond to the unpredictability of unscheduled care. Whilst other elements focus on the up-to-date management of neurosurgical conditions, this Element aims to provide context on the evolution of delivering emergency surgical care in the western world.

Unscheduled Care

Delivering clinically effective and cost-effective unscheduled care is a key cornerstone of any healthcare system and requires significant resources and dovetailing of services to deliver optimal outcomes. Emergency and urgent care fall under the bracket of unscheduled care and can be considered as any illness or accident requiring medical attention immediately or within 24 hours, respectively (1). This requires a reactive component to a healthcare service (2) and can have a detrimental impact on other aspects of healthcare, particularly the consistent delivery of elective care.

Healthcare policy aims to introduce and maintain proactive and preventative measures that improve the care of long-term conditions in the community. Despite this, exacerbations of chronic conditions and the natural history of de novo conditions presenting acutely continue to necessitate unscheduled admissions to hospital.

The Evolving Nature of Emergency Surgery

The management of the unscheduled component of a surgical workload has had to progressively evolve, from strategic reorganisation of services to changing the delivery of care at the coalface. Several publications have highlighted deficiencies and issues prompting changes in the delivery of care.

Reorganisation of Services: Trauma Networks

The management of trauma has made considerable progress. The USA generated evidence during the latter half of the twentieth century that rationalising trauma care into trauma networks reduced mortality (3). Trauma networks consist of a hub-and-spoke model with a central major trauma centre (MTC) and surrounding feeder hospitals (trauma units). This concentrates surgical and critical care facilities and expertise alongside the development of pre-hospital triage and inter-hospital transfer protocols (4).

Reports in the 1990s and early 2000s emphasised regional variation and substandard levels of trauma care provided across the UK (5,6), alongside raising concerns regarding the management of traumatic brain injury (TBI) (7) and neurosurgical intensive care bed availability (8). The report 'Trauma, Who Cares?' (9) highlighted concerns on trauma care to the public, politicians and the medical professionals, prompting the past decade of standardising and improving trauma care in the UK.

In 2012, 26 Regional Trauma Networks were rolled out across England (10). Since their introduction, nationwide improvements in outcomes have been reported by the Trauma Audit and Research Network (TARN) (11). Other examples of networks in the National Health Service (NHS) exist, including Regional Spinal Networks and the current development of Integrated Stroke Delivery Networks.

Trauma and Emergency Surgery Courses

The direct provision of surgical care has made considerable strides. Courses have been devised focusing on the initial assessment and management of trauma (i.e. Advanced Trauma and Life Support (ATLS) and European Trauma Course (ETC)) and the development of non-cadaveric and cadaveric simulators focusing on improving surgical skills, including the introduction of boot camps throughout surgical training.

The origins of ATLS are steeped in tragedy. In 1976, an orthopaedic surgeon in the USA was piloting a small plane with his family on board that crashed in the Nebraska countryside (12). Their experience demonstrated deficiencies in trauma care, prompting the development of the ATLS course. In 2006, the ETC was introduced to cater to the European experience of trauma (13).

Within the NHS, there are concerns on the extent of operative exposure encountered throughout training. The causes are multifaceted, relating to changes in workforce numbers, statutory legislation limiting working hours and changes in the surgical management of conditions (i.e. endovascular coiling rather than clipping of intracranial aneurysms) (14). The use of cadaveric and non-cadaveric models to develop and improve surgical skills has been gaining traction. Live models for developing real-time surgical skills and competence in traumatic and non-traumatic emergency pathologies have demonstrated their benefit (15–17). Surgical simulators, veering away from classical cadaveric models, have been devised for neurosurgery, yet their efficacy and availability remains unclear (18). The benefit of simulators extends beyond the acquisition of technical skills and extends to the development of non-operative technical skills such as decision-making, communication and teamwork (14).

Boot camps for surgical registrars have been widely accepted, permitting the standardised delivery of knowledge and technical skills to trainees at various points throughout training. Improvements in clinical skills, knowledge and confidence have been demonstrated (19,20).

The Emergence of Emergency Surgery as a Specialty

The nature of certain surgical specialties has evolved with the specialty of emergency surgery being increasingly recognised. In 2003, acute care surgery (ACS) emerged as a dedicated surgical sub-specialty in the USA in response to an increasing surgical workload, sub-specialisation and the decline in expertise for managing acute non-traumatic emergencies (21). Evidence has demonstrated improved morbidity and mortality with ACS (22). In the USA, ACS has expanded to include emergency surgery, trauma surgery and critical care services with a dedicated surgical team providing this service distinct from other surgical services.

In the UK, a variant of ACS has emerged: emergency general surgery (EGS). Emergency general surgery aims to reduce the impact on elective care provision and tackle the increasing difficulty in providing a 'generalist' service (23). Unlike the USA, the provision of EGS is solely related to non-traumatic emergency surgery and predominantly focuses on intra-abdominal pathology and relies on intensive care physicians to deliver critical care services. Despite the lack of a dedicated training pathway, EGS specialists and units do exist (24).

The physical separation of emergency surgical care from elective care has not been limited to general surgery and was recommended to improve the delivery of care and improve efficiency, teaching and patient outcomes (25). Similar approaches have occurred within neurosurgery. A new diagnosis of a brain tumour, having previously been managed as an emergency hospital admission, is increasingly managed via an urgent elective pathway with some units in the UK using day-case admissions for biopsies and resections (26).

Key Reports Changing the Delivery of Emergency Surgery

Within the UK, regulatory and commissioning bodies have produced reports, standards, policies and guidelines determining the organisation of services and providing recommendations for the management of neurosurgical pathologies. In the following, we focus specifically on the National Confidential Enquiry into Patient Outcome and Death (NCEPOD) and the Getting It Right First Time (GIRFT) programmes.

NCEPOD is an independent organisation aiming to maintain and improve standards of healthcare across all medical and surgical specialties and publishes its reports online (https://www.ncepod.org.uk/). Early reports from NCEPOD focused on peri-operative care and had seismic impacts on the delivery of emergency surgery and trauma care. The two reports, Who Operates When 1 (27) and 2 (28) provided a stark insight into the delivery surgical care and prompted discussions on when and who should be performing surgery, and resulted in the categorisation of interventions (see Table 1). Other reports consider the care of trauma patients (9), high-risk surgical patients (29), emergency surgery in the elderly (30,31) and those with aneurysmal subarachnoid haemorrhage (32).

The Getting It Right First Time programme was devised to formally evaluate all providers of a specialty within England, aiming to reduce variations in practice and promote best practice in all aspects of care. Initially conducted in orthopaedic surgery, it has been conducted for cranial neurosurgery (33) and spinal surgery (34) with paediatric neurosurgery being currently under review and a re-review of cranial neurosurgery to be published shortly.

Emergency Neurosurgery

Emergency neurosurgery can be considered as any neurosurgical condition that progresses rapidly requiring specialist intervention to minimise further damage to the neuraxis. It encompasses all aspects of adult and paediatric cranial and spinal sub-specialties, including the post-operative management of elective complications.

The Burden of Emergency Neurosurgical Disease

Worldwide, approximately 22.6 million people per year develop a neurosurgical disorder that requires the input of a neurosurgeon, with 13.8 million requiring operative intervention. The bulk of the workload consists of TBI (45%), cerebrovascular accidents (20%), hydrocephalus (7%) and brain tumours (5%). There is worldwide disparity in providing neurosurgical care as 80% of cases are estimated to arise in low- and middle-income countries whilst 44% of neurosurgeons work in high-income countries (35).

Within the UK, the data on the extent of emergency surgical care remains incomplete and inconsistent with estimates of emergency admissions comprising 40–50% of the pan-specialty surgical workload.

In 2018/2019, NHS Digital identified a total of 5,269,703 pan-surgical admissions in England. Considerable variation exists in the number of admissions, proportion of emergency admissions and the total workload (see Table 2). Neurosurgery accounts for 1.7% of the total surgical workload, and 27.2% of its admissions in 2018/2019 were emergencies (36). From 2000 to 2019, the

Table 1 NCEPOD categorisation of intervention

Code	Category	Definition	Example	Timing
1	Immediate	Immediate (1A) life or (1B) limb or organ saving intervention. Simultaneously performed with resuscitation	Ruptured AAA. Craniotomy for evacuation of ASDH	Within minutes of operative decision
2	Urgent	Intervention for acute onset OR clinical deterioration of potentially life-threatening conditions; OR for conditions that may threaten the survival of a limb or organ; OR fixation of fractures; OR relief of distressing symptoms	Fixation of neck of femur fracture	Within hours of operative decision
3	Expedited	Stable patient requiring early treatment where the condition is not an immediate threat to life, limb or organ	Excision of tumour with potential to bleed or obstruct	Within days of operative decision
4	Elective	Intervention planned or booked in advance of routine admission to hospital	Total hip replacement. Lumbar microdiscectomy for radiculopathy	Timing to suit patient, staff and hospital

Table 2 Data obtained from Hospital Episode Statistics (NHS Digital) displaying the number of admissions for each surgical specialty in 2018/2019

Specialty	Total admissions (*n*)	Emergency admissions (*n*)	Emergency admissions (%)	Proportion of surgical workload (%)
General surgery	1,842,329	714,528	38.8%	35.0%
Urology	660,492	129,009	19.5%	3.9%
Trauma and orthopaedics	1,108,408	294,205	26.5%	21.0%
Otorhinolaryngology	343,537	87,311	25.4%	6.5%
Ophthalmology	733,880	15,195	2.1%	13.9%
Oral and maxillo-facial surgery	99,960	14,652	14.7%	1.9%
Neurosurgery	90,144	24,533	27.2%	1.7%
Plastic surgery	267,450	59,134	22.1%	5.1%
Cardiothoracic surgery	62,078	8,701	14.0%	1.2%
Paediatric surgery	61,425	17,257	28.1%	1.2%
All surgical specialties	**5,269,703**	**1,364,525**	**25.9%**	**100%**
All hospital admissions	**17,127,498**	**6,437,959**	**37.6%**	

Considerable variation across the surgical specialties in the proportion of their emergency admissions and total surgical workload is displayed.

number of emergency and total neurosurgical admissions rose by 85% and 87%, respectively. Wahba *et al.* (2022) identified 371,418 adult neurosurgical admissions in England between 2013 and 2018, with 77.3% of cases receiving a primary neurosurgical procedure and 39% of these total admissions being unscheduled (37). Since the COVID-19 pandemic in early 2020 until the time of writing, the total number of neurosurgical admissions has decreased by 30% whilst emergency admissions have only reduced by 2% (38).

Neurosurgery in Specific Countries

Emergency neurosurgery in the UK and the Republic of Ireland is provided by nationally funded services that are available to all, free at the point of access; however, other models of care exist in Europe and the USA. We provide an overview of services provided within the UK, Republic of Ireland, the Netherlands and the USA.

United Kingdom and the Republic of Ireland

The UK and the Republic of Ireland has 36 publicly funded centres that provide paediatric and adult emergency and elective neurosurgical services. Privately funded neurosurgical services exist, but they do not provide emergency services.

England

In England, 150 NHS Trusts deliver healthcare to approximately 56.5 million people, with 30 Trusts providing adult and paediatric neurosurgical services. Twenty-four units deliver adult neurosurgery with 16 units providing a solely adult service and 8 units providing a combined adult and paediatric service (Table 3). Twenty-two of these units are co-located with an MTC emphasising the close relationship between major trauma and neurosurgical trauma. The catchment population size per unit varies between 1 and 3.5 million people. In 2020, there were 453 consultant neurosurgeons in the UK and Ireland (39). Inpatient capacity ranges widely from 22 to 96 beds. The number of non-elective procedures performed across the 24 adult units ranged between 200 and 800 per year (33). Some units have a dedicated emergency neurosurgery theatre that can help minimise the impact on elective operating.

The provision of cranial and spinal services varies between neurosurgical units with an increasing trend towards the separation of cranial and spinal rotas. A spinal service within a single hospital may be cross-covered by in-house neurosurgical and orthopaedic departments. Forty NHS Trusts are designated as specialist providers of adult spinal surgery and paediatric spinal surgery is delivered by 24 NHS Trusts (34).

Table 3 Thirty providers of neurosurgical services in England

Adult services	Combined adult and paediatric services	Paediatric services
Barking, Havering, and Redbridge University Hospitals NHS Trust	Cambridge University Hospitals NHS Foundation Trust King's College Hospital NHS Foundation Trust	Alder Hey Children's NHS Foundation Trust
Barts Health NHS Trust		Birmingham Women's and Children's Hospital NHS Foundation Trust
Brighton and Sussex University Hospitals NHS Trust	Leeds Teaching Hospitals NHS Trust	
Hull University Teaching Hospitals NHS Trust	Newcastle Hospitals NHS Foundation Trust	Great Ormond Street Hospital NHS Foundation Trust
Imperial College Healthcare NHS Trust	Nottingham University Hospitals NHS Trust	
Lancashire Teaching Hospitals NHS Trust		
North Bristol NHS Trust		
Northern Care Alliance NHS Foundation Trust	Oxford University Hospitals NHS Foundation Trust	Manchester University NHS Foundation Trust
Sheffield Teaching Hospitals NHS Foundation Trust	St George's University Hospitals NHS Foundation Trust	Sheffield Children's Hospital NHS Foundation Trust
South Tees Hospitals NHS Foundation Trust	University Hospital Southampton NHS Foundation Trust	University Hospitals Bristol NHS Foundation Trust
The Walton Centre NHS Foundation Trust		
University College London Hospitals NHS Foundation Trust		
University Hospital Coventry and Warwickshire NHS Trust		
University Hospitals Birmingham NHS Foundation Trust		
University Hospitals Plymouth NHS Trust		
University Hospitals of North Midlands NHS Trust		

Certain units have dedicated vascular, paediatric, general neurosurgery and spine on call rotas. Within the UK, the method of urgently or emergently referring to neurosurgery has altered with the progressive implementation of electronic referral systems. This has permitted significant improvements in prioritising workload, improving the quality of documentation and increasing the speed of responsiveness (40). The requirement for direct communication in-person or over the telephone in emergent situations continues to exist.

Paediatric neurosurgery is a low-volume, high-risk and high-cost specialty with a high emergency workload. Its optimal delivery remains a source of ongoing debate, with concerns around the rationalisation of services, maximising outcomes and maintaining adequate case exposure whilst trying to maintain services near people's homes. There are 14 units that provide paediatric neurosurgery in England, of which 6 are standalone paediatric units and 8 units deliver a combined paediatric and adult neurosurgery service. Thirteen units are co-located with an MTC.

Since 1988, the British Paediatric Neurosurgery Group has strived for the development of paediatric neurosurgery as a dedicated sub-specialty and to promote high standards of care for children. At the turn of the twenty-first century, the Public Enquiry into Children's Heart Surgery identified significant concerns on the delivery of paediatric cardiothoracic surgery prompting a raft of changes on paediatric care across the NHS (41). A task force was formed by the Society of British Neurological Surgeons to determine the minimum requirements of a safe paediatric neurosurgery service, resulting in the publication of two reports: Safe Paediatric Neurosurgery (42) and Safe Paediatric Neurosurgery 2001 (43). Despite this, controversy continued (44–46) and is summarised in a review article by Young (47).

Service specifications devised by NHS England exist for adult neurosurgery (48), paediatric neurosurgery (49) and complex spine surgery (50). These define the minimum operational requirements for each service to remain commissioned.

Scotland

Neurosurgical services are delivered in four cities in Scotland, providing care for approximately 5.5 million inhabitants (see Table 4). Spinal surgery is provided by the four neurosurgical services and co-located orthopaedic departments as well as a fifth orthopaedic unit in Inverness. The Scottish Trauma Network supports four regional trauma networks and the Scottish Ambulance Service. Each regional network submits their data to the Scottish Trauma Audit Group, the equivalent of TARN in England.

Table 4 The cities of Scotland containing neurosurgical centres and their overseeing regional health board

City	Regional Health Board	Population (%)	Adult hospital	Paediatric hospital
Edinburgh	NHS Lothian	867,000 (17.1%)	RHCYP and DCN[a]	Royal Hospital for Sick Children
Glasgow	NHS GG&C	2,700,000 (53.3%)	The Queen Elizabeth University Hospital	Royal Hospital for Children
Aberdeen	NHS Grampian	800,000 (15.8%)	Aberdeen Royal Infirmary	Royal Aberdeen Children Hospital
Dundee	NHS Tayside	700,000 (13.8%)	Ninewells Hospital	Tayside Children's Hospital

[a] The Royal Hospital for Children and Young People (RHCYP) and the Department of Clinical Neurosciences (DCN) provide paediatric and adult neurosurgery services based *at* a new hospital in Little France, Edinburgh. The DCN had been previously located at the Western General Hospital in Edinburgh.

The Managed Service Network (MSN) for Neurosurgery is a collaboration between the Scottish neurosurgical centres, which was commenced in 2009. The MSN is designed to permit the neurosurgical centres to function as a single service and facilitate teamwork, improving and defining standards of care, auditing clinical practice, workforce planning and supporting the national training programme. The MSN has categorised different forms of paediatric neurosurgery that should be undertaken in the various paediatric centres, partly reflected by the requirement for post-operative intensive care, as well as the rarity of the procedure and centralising expertise (51).

Wales

The provision of neurosurgical services in Wales is divided geographically. In South- and Mid-Wales (approximately 2.5 million people), adult and paediatric emergency and elective neurosurgery is provided by the University Hospital of Wales and the Noah's Ark Children's Hospital, overseen by the Cardiff and Vale University Health Board. Spinal surgery services are also provided at Moriston Hospital, Swansea. In North Wales (approximately 700,000 persons), adults and children are referred to the Walton Centre and Alder Hey Children's Hospital in Liverpool, respectively. Trauma networks exist in Wales, with North Wales covered by the North Wales Major Trauma Network and various English trauma networks bordering with Wales. The South Wales Trauma Network was launched in 2020 with University Hospital of Wales acting as the MTC.

Northern Ireland

In Northern Ireland, the Royal Victoria Hospital and Royal Belfast Hospital for Sick Children, Belfast provide adult and paediatric elective and emergency services to approximately 1.8 million people. The Northern Ireland Major Trauma Network was established in 2017 and the Royal Victoria Hospital is the designated MTC. Health and social care services are managed by Health and Social Care with overall responsibility lying with the Department of Health.

Republic of Ireland

Three neurosurgical departments provide a service for the 5.1 million people residing within the Republic of Ireland:

- National Neurosurgical Centre at Beaumont Hospital, Dublin;
- Department of Paediatric Neurosurgery, Dublin;
- Cork University Hospital (CUH).

Beaumont Hospital is a large academic teaching hospital providing a broad range of services to the local population and acts as the national referral centre for neurosurgery and neurology. The Department of Paediatric Neurosurgery provides national emergency and elective services, including craniofacial surgery. The Munster province (population of approximately one million) is served by CUH although certain neurosurgical cases may be transferred from CUH to Beaumont Hospital. The development and implementation of a trauma network within Ireland is underway (52) with CUH and The Mater Hospital (Dublin) being chosen as the MTCs for Ireland. The latter assignment provides controversy as it does not have a co-located neurosurgical unit.

United States of America

The provision of emergency neurosurgery services in the USA is diverse, especially when compared to countries with more uniform healthcare systems, such as the UK. This is partly explained by the enormity of the country comprising different states with different laws and fiscal policies governing healthcare delivery and the absence of a uniform hospital or practice type found in the USA (53).

Despite this variation, certain Federal laws and standards set out by national bodies must be met to deliver certain emergency neurosurgery services (54). The American College of Surgeons Committee on Trauma verifies and designates hospitals as trauma centres and sets standards on where neurosurgery trauma should be managed. Approximately 500 hospitals fulfil the criteria to be a level 1 or 2 trauma centre (55). These centres are required to have neurosurgery coverage 24/7/365. Once a hospital is designated as a trauma centre, emergency medical services (EMSs) will triage patients and bring them to the closest and most appropriate emergency department. The EMSs play a key role in determining which hospital to transfer their trauma patients and where neurosurgeons will receive their referrals.

Occasionally, multiple trauma centres in a single area are 'in competition' for patients. However, multiple patients from a single trauma incident are frequently taken to different trauma centres to avoid overwhelming a single department (54).

Unlike the UK, neurosurgeons are major providers of endovascular interventions for emergency stroke services. Stroke centres have national consensus guidelines for the acute treatment of stroke and must be certified by nationally recognised bodies (54). The availability of a neurosurgeon is a necessity for a hospital to achieve primary stroke centre certification, with even more stringent requirements for a comprehensive stroke centre designation.

Geographic proximity and the availability of neurosurgical services are the main guiding factors determining patient transfer, but a patient's medical insurance status can also play a role. If two equally good choices exist for transfer, their insurance or affiliation with a hospital may ultimately determine their destination. However, the Emergency Medical Treatment and Labor Act mandates anyone coming to an emergency department to be stabilised and treated, regardless of insurance status or the ability to pay (56). In serious neurosurgical emergencies, providing insurance or hospital affiliation information is often hampered and the patient would be transferred to the nearest specialised centre.

The growth of specialised centres and the increasing litigious environment have made it increasingly difficult for smaller neurosurgery practices to deliver emergency neurosurgery. Hospitals are increasingly employing large neurosurgical groups who are salaried with their contracts including the provision of emergency call coverage.

Given the scale of the USA, geographical inequity exists for neurosurgery emergency provision (57). The majority of trauma and stroke centres are in urban areas with vast rural areas being without easy access to these specialised centres delaying access to definitive care.

The Netherlands

The Netherlands has a population of approximately 17.4 million people and neurosurgery is provided by approximately 150 neurosurgeons affiliated with 13 neurosurgical centres and 4 hospital partnerships. Regionalisation has occurred with the existence of stroke and trauma centres. Since 1999, the Netherlands is organised into 11 trauma regions, with each region having a single level 1 trauma centre that provides emergency neurosurgery (58,59). Certain aspects of neurosurgery, such as paediatrics, are increasingly supra-regionalised.

The point of entry for neurosurgery referrals is the neurosurgery resident on call. However, departmental consultants or neurology residents may act as the first tier for centres without a neurosurgery resident. A second tier can exist with specialists in spinal or vascular neurosurgery being available when required.

The mechanism for funding healthcare in the Netherlands is unlike the UK or the USA. A statutory obligation is placed on all residents to have basic insurance that provides access to a standard level of services.

Conclusion

Providing unscheduled care is a fundamental component of any healthcare system and forms a significant part of a neurosurgeon's workload. Alongside improving our understanding and management of disease processes, we must

Table 5 Ideal characteristics of a healthcare system providing emergency surgery to a population

Workforce and service delivery	• Optimal number of faculty and trainees to minimise onerous on call rota duties and maximise service delivery and fulfil training requirements
	• Dedicated specialty opinion and surgical expertise consistently available
	• Maintaining adequate operative cases to maintain skills and expertise
	• Equal and equitable access to services with minimal geographical variation
Infrastructure	• Dedicated emergency theatre and inpatient facilities to prevent disruption and delays to elective services
	• Redundancy within the system to allow for fluctuations in workload
	• Access to relevant allied medical and surgical specialties including neuro-rehabilitation facilities
	• Inter-hospital agreements for transfer
	• Closely located to people's homes with adequate facilities for relatives (particularly for paediatric cases)
	• Close and reciprocal links with:
	○ research and educational institutions to maximise the development of new knowledge and the training of future clinicians
	○ industry for the development and usage of novel surgical technologies
	○ primary and emergency care and public health systems
Governance and information management	• Real-time auditing of surgical outcomes and patient-reported outcome measures
	• Consistent and reliable referral systems and electronic health records

aim to optimise the delivery of clinically effective and cost-effective unscheduled care. The introduction of trauma networks has been a success in improving patient outcomes; however, we should continue to maintain momentum in developing new and existing models of care.

Ideally, a Utopian system with a minimal financial cost should exist, yet what that system would consist of and how it could be achieved remain unanswered. It may contain some of the following characteristics (see Table 5). The enormity of the task at hand is aptly put into perspective by Arneja and Buchel (60) when considering the high number of requirements for a single operation to occur:

- Aligned patient variables (correct indication, consent, fasted and optimised physiology)
- Suitable infrastructure (inter-hospital transport, pre-operative, operative and post-operative)
- Appropriate equipment
- Adequate staffing (surgeon, anaesthetist, intensivist, nursing and support staff).

Despite this, it remains prudent to stay motivated and open-minded for developing this optimal system and a collaborative approach is essential within the field of neurosurgery, learning from the experiences of other specialties and between nations.

References

1. O'Cathain A, Knowles E, Munro J, Nicholl J. Exploring the effect of changes to service provision on the use of unscheduled care in England: population surveys. BMC Health Serv Res. 27 April 2007;7:61.
2. Pines JM, Lotrecchiano GR, Zocchi MS, et al. A conceptual model for episodes of acute, unscheduled care. Ann Emerg Med. October 2016;68 (4):484–491.e3.
3. Nathens AB, Jurkovich GJ, Rivara FP, Maier RV. Effectiveness of state trauma systems in reducing injury-related mortality: a national evaluation. J Trauma. January 2000;48(1):25–30; discussion 30–1.
4. Metcalfe D, Perry DC, Bouamra O, et al. Regionalisation of trauma care in England. Bone Joint J. September 2016;98-B(9):1253–61.
5. Saleh M. Commission on the provision of surgical services. The management of patients with major injuries. Ann R Coll Surg Engl. July 1989; 71(4 Suppl):58.
6. Browne J, Coats TJ, Lloyd DA, et al. High quality acute care for the severely injured is not consistently available in England, Wales and Northern Ireland: report of a survey by the Trauma Committee, The Royal College of Surgeons of England. Ann R Coll Surg Engl. March 2006;88(2):103–7.
7. McKeating EG, Andrews PJ, Tocher JI, Menon DK. The intensive care of severe head injury: a survey of non-neurosurgical centres in the United Kingdom. Br J Neurosurg. February 1998;12(1):7–14.
8. Crimmins DW, Palmer JD. Snapshot view of emergency neurosurgical head injury care in Great Britain and Ireland. J Neurol Neurosurg Psychiatry. January 2000;68(1):8–13.
9. NCEPOD. Trauma: Who Cares? NCEPOD; 2007.
10. McCullough AL, Haycock JC, Forward DP, Moran CG. Major trauma networks in England. Br J Anaesth. 1 August 2014;113(2):202–6.
11. Moran CG, Lecky F, Bouamra O, et al. Changing the system – major trauma patients and their outcomes in the NHS (England) 2008–17. EClinicalMedicine. August 2018;2–3:13–21.
12. Styner JK. The birth of advanced trauma life support (ATLS). Surgeon. July 2006;4(3):163–5.
13. Thies K, Gwinnutt C, Driscoll P, et al. The European Trauma Course – from concept to course. Resuscitation. July 2007;74(1):135–41.
14. Nicholas R, Humm G, MacLeod KE, et al. Simulation in surgical training: prospective cohort study of access, attitudes and experiences of surgical trainees in the UK and Ireland. Int J Surg. July 2019;67:94–100.

15. Gaarder C, Naess PA, Buanes T, Pillgram-Larsen J. Advanced surgical trauma care training with a live porcine model. Injury. June 2005;36(6):718–24.

16. Shannon AH, Cullen JM, Dahl JJ, et al. Porcine model of infrarenal abdominal aortic aneurysm. J Vis Exp [Internet]. 21 November 2019; (153). http://dx.doi.org/10.3791/60169.

17. Guenther TM, Chen SA, Gustafson JD, Wozniak CJ, Kiaii B. Development of a porcine model of emergency resternotomy at a low-volume cardiac surgery centre. Interact Cardiovasc Thorac Surg. 7 December 2020;31(6):803–5.

18. Davids J, Manivannan S, Darzi A, et al. Simulation for skills training in neurosurgery: a systematic review, meta-analysis, and analysis of progressive scholarly acceptance. Neurosurg Rev. August 2021;44(4):1853–67.

19. Blackmore C, Austin J, Lopushinsky SR, Donnon T. Effects of postgraduate medical education 'boot camps' on clinical skills, knowledge, and confidence: a meta-analysis. J Grad Med Educ. December 2014;6(4):643–52.

20. Singh P, Aggarwal R, Pucher PH, et al. An immersive 'simulation week' enhances clinical performance of incoming surgical interns improved performance persists at 6 months follow-up. Surgery. March 2015;157(3):432–43.

21. van der Wee MJL, van der Wilden G, Hoencamp R. Acute care surgery models worldwide: a systematic review. World J Surg. August 2020;44 (8):2622–37.

22. Chana P, Burns EM, Arora S, Darzi AW, Faiz OD. A systematic review of the impact of dedicated emergency surgical services on patient outcomes. Ann Surg. January 2016;263(1):20–7.

23. Ramsay G, Wohlgemut JM, Jansen JO. Emergency general surgery in the United Kingdom: a lot of general, not many emergencies, and not much surgery. J Trauma Acute Care Surg. September 2018;85(3):500–6.

24. Bokhari S, Walsh U, Qurashi K, et al. Impact of a dedicated emergency surgical unit on early laparoscopic cholecystectomy for acute cholecystitis. Ann R Coll Surg Engl. February 2016;98(2):107–15.

25. Royal College of Surgeons (England). Separating Emergency and Elective Surgical Care: Recommendations for Practice. Royal College of Surgeons of England; 2007.

26. Grundy PL, Weidmann C, Bernstein M. Day-case neurosurgery for brain tumours: the early United Kingdom experience. Br J Neurosurg. June 2008;22(3):360–7.

27. NCEPOD. Who Operates When? (I) [Internet]. NCEPOD; 1997 Sep [cited 8 February 2022]. www.ncepod.org.uk/1995_6.html.

28. NCEPOD. Who Operates When? (II) [Internet]. NCEPOD; November 2003. www.ncepod.org.uk/2003wow.html.

29. NCEPOD. Peri-operative Care: Knowing the Risk. NCEPOD; 2011.

30. NCEPOD. Extremes of Age. NCEPOD; 1999.

31. NCEPOD. Elective & Emergency Surgery in the Elderly: An Age Old Problem. NCEPOD; 2010.

32. NCEPOD. Managing the Flow? NCEPOD; 2013.

33. GIRFT. Cranial Neurosurgery. GIRFT Programme National Specialty Report. NHS Improvement; 2018.

34. GIRFT. Spinal Services. GIRFT Programme National Specialty Report. NHS Improvement; 2019.

35. Dewan MC, Rattani A, Fieggen G, et al. Global neurosurgery: the current capacity and deficit in the provision of essential neurosurgical care. Executive Summary of the Global Neurosurgery Initiative at the Program in Global Surgery and Social Change. J Neurosurg. 1 April 2018;1–10.

36. NHS Digital. Hospital Admitted Patient Care Activity 2018–2019 [Internet]. NHS Digital. 2019 [cited 2 August 2022]. https://digital.nhs.uk/data-and-information/publications/statistical/hospital-admitted-patient-care-activity/2018-19.

37. Wahba, A.J., Cromwell, D.A., Hutchinson, P.J., Mathew, R.K., and Phillips, N. 2022. Mortality as an indicator of quality of neurosurgical care in England: a retrospective cohort study. *BMJ* Open, 12: e067409.

38. NHS Digital. Hospital Admitted Patient Care Activity [Internet]. NHS Digital. 2021 [cited 10 February 2022]. https://digital.nhs.uk/data-and-information/publications/statistical/hospital-admitted-patient-care-activity.

39. Whitehouse K, Sinha S, Thomson S, Jenkins A. UK Neurosurgery Workforce Report. Society of British Neurological Surgeons; 2020.

40. Matloob SA, Hyam JA, Thorne L, Bradford R. Improving neurosurgical communication and reducing risk and registrar burden using a novel online database referral platform. Br J Neurosurg. 22 March 2016;30(2):191–4.

41. Department of Health. The report of the public inquiry into children's heart surgery at the Bristol Royal Infirmary 1984–1995: learning from Bristol [Internet]. Department of Health; 2001. https://webarchive.nationalarchives.gov.uk/ukgwa/20090811143810/www.bristol-inquiry.org.uk/final_report/report/index.htm.

42. SBNS. Safe Paediatric Neurosurgery. SBNS; 1998.

43. SBNS. Safe Paediatric Neurosurgery 2001. SBNS; 2001.

44. Chumas P, Pople I, Mallucci C, Steers J, Crimmins D. British paediatric neurosurgery – a time for change? Br J Neurosurg. December 2008;22(6): 719–28.

45. Mitchell P. Future UK paediatric neurosurgery. Br J Neurosurg. February 2010;24(1):3–4; discussion 5–7.

46. Mallucci C, Thompson D. Safe and sustainable British paediatric neurosurgery – 1 year on and where are we now? A response to 'Future UK paediatric neurosurgery'. Br J Neurosurg. 1 February 2010;24(1):5–6.

47. Young AE. Designing a safe and sustainable pediatric neurosurgical practice: the English experience. Paediatr Anaesth. July 2014;24(7): 649–56.

48. NHS England. Service Specification: Neurosurgery (Adults). NHS England; 2019.

49. NHS England. Service Specification: Paediatric Neurosurgery Services. NHS England; 2013.

50. NHS England. Service Specification: Complex Spine Surgery Services (All Ages). NHS England; 2021.

51. MSN. Paediatric Neurosurgical Procedures. Managed Service Network for Neurosurgery; 2020.

52. Department of Health. A Trauma System: Report of the Trauma Steering Group for Ireland [Internet]. Department of Health; June 2018. www.gov.ie/en/publication/c8640e-a-trauma-system-for-ireland-report-of-the-trauma-steering-group/?referrer=www.health.gov.ie/wp-content/uploads/2018/02/Report-of-the-Trauma-Steering-Group-A-Trauma-System-for-Ireland.pdf.

53. Babu MA, Stroink AR, Timmons SD, Orrico KO, Prall JA. Neurosurgical coverage for emergency and trauma call. Neurosurgery. 1 April 2019;84 (4):977–84.

54. Wang HE, Yealy DM. Distribution of specialized care centers in the United States. Ann Emerg Med. November 2012;60(5):632–637.e7.

55. American Hospital Association. Fast Facts on U.S. Hospitals, 2022 [Internet]. American Hospital Association. 2022 [cited 6 May 2022]. www.aha.org/statistics/fast-facts-us-hospitals.

56. American College of Emergency Physicians. EMTALA Fact Sheet [Internet]. 2022 [cited 6 May 2022]. www.acep.org/life-as-a-physician/ethics–legal/emtala/emtala-fact-sheet/.

57. Branas CC, MacKenzie EJ, Williams JC, et al. Access to trauma centers in the United States. JAMA. 1 June 2005;293(21):2626–33.

58. Landelijk Netwerk Acute Zorg. Landelijke Traumaregistratie [Internet]. 2021 [cited 5 December 2022]. www.lnaz.nl/cms/files/rapportage-2020-nl-rectificatie.pdf.

59. Hietbrink F, Houwert RM, van Wessem KJP, et al. The evolution of trauma care in the Netherlands over 20 years. Eur J Trauma Emerg Surg. April 2020;46(2):329–35.

60. Arneja JS, Buchel EW. Does the ideal health care system exist? Will it be accepted in Canada? Plast Surg (Oakv). 2014 Spring;22(1):7–8.

Cambridge Elements ☰

Emergency Neurosurgery

Nihal Gurusinghe
Lancashire Teaching Hospital NHS Trust

Professor Nihal Gurusinghe is a Consultant Neurosurgeon at the Lancashire Teaching Hospitals NHS Trust. He is on the Executive Council of the Society of British Neurological Surgeons as the Lead for NICE (National Institute for Health and Care Excellence) guidelines relating to neurosurgical practice. He is also an examiner for the UK and International FRCS examinations in Neurosurgery.

Peter Hutchinson
University of Cambridge, Society of British Neurological Surgeons and Royal College of Surgeons of England

Peter Hutchinson BSc MBBS FFSEM FRCS(SN) PhD FMedSci is Professor of Neurosurgery and Head of the Division of Academic Neurosurgery at the University of Cambridge, and Honorary Consultant Neurosurgeon at Addenbrooke's Hospital. He is Director of Clinical Research at the Royal College of Surgeons of England and Meetings Secretary of the Society of British Neurological Surgeons.

Ioannis Fouyas
Royal College of Surgeons of Edinburgh

Ioannis Fouyas is a Consultant Neurosurgeon in Edinburgh. His clinical interests focus on the treatment of complex cerebrovascular and skull base pathologies. His academic endeavours concentrate in the field of cerebrovascular pathophysiology. His passion is technical surgical training, fulfilled in collaboration with the Royal College of Surgeons of Edinburgh. Finally, he pursues Undergraduate Neuroscience teaching, with a particular focus on functional Neuroanatomy.

Naomi Slator
North Bristol NHS Trust

Naomi Slator FRCS (SN) is a Consultant Spinal Neurosurgeon based at North Bristol NHS Trust. She has a specialist interest in Complex Spine alongside Cranial and Spinal Trauma. She completed her neurosurgical training in Birmingham and a six-month Fellowship in CSF and Trauma (2019). She then went on to complete her Spinal Fellowship in Leeds (2020) before moving to the southwest to take up her consultant post.

Ian Kamaly-Asl
Royal Manchester Children's Hospital

Ian Kamaly-Asl is a full time paediatric neurosurgeon and Honorary Chair at Royal Manchester Children's Hospital. He trained in North Western Deanery with fellowships at Boston Children's Hospital and Sick Kids in Toronto. Ian is a member of council of The Royal College of Surgeons of England and The SBNS where he is lead for mentoring and tackling oppressive behaviours.

Peter Whitfield
University Hospitals Plymouth NHS Trust

Professor Peter Whitfield is a Consultant Neurosurgeon at the South West Neurosurgical Centre, University Hospitals Plymouth NHS Trust. His clinical interests include vascular neurosurgery, neuro oncology and trauma. He has held many roles in postgraduate neurosurgical education and is President of the Society of British Neurological Surgeons. Peter has published widely, and is passionate about education, training and the promotion of clinical research.

About the Series

Elements in Emergency Neurosurgery is intended for trainees and practitioners in Neurosurgery and Emergency Medicine as well as allied specialties all over the world. Authored by international experts, this series provides core knowledge, common clinical pathways and recommendations on the management of acute conditions of the brain and spine.

Cambridge Elements ☰

Emergency Neurosurgery

Elements in the Series

The Challenges of On-Call Neurosurgery
Abteen Mostofi, Marco Lee and Nihal Gurusinghe

Mild Traumatic Brain Injury including Concussion
Thomas D. Parker and Colette Griffin

Models for Delivering High Quality Emergency Neurosurgery in High Income Countries
Matthew A. Boissaud-Cooke, Marike Broekman, Jeroen van Dijck, Marco Lee and Paul Grundy

A full series listing is available at: www.cambridge.org/EEMN